TRACKS
From Fake to Fabulous

Embracing the God Given Me

A Portion of the Proceeds from this book will go towards
EDUCATING, EMPOWERING and UPLIFTING young
black women to embrace Beauty from the Inside Out

Lisa Simpson Hoover

3G Publishing, Inc.
Loganville, GA 30052
www.3gpublishinginc.com
Phone: 1-888-442-9637

First published by 3G Publishing, Inc. May, 2015
ISBN: 978-1-941247-00-6
Printed in the United States of America

Contents

Dedication

This book is dedicated to my mother, the late Loraine Coles Simpson. She is the wind beneath my wings.

A special thanks to my husband Robert for planting the seed to write this book. He validates it.

I lead by example for my niece Vivian Loraine and daughters, Lena, Lyric and Annica.

My desire. A world where girls and women despite the color of their skin or eyes, shape of their lips or derriere, length of their hair, or fullness or lack of breast, embrace and appreciate their authenticity inside out.

The Author

Lisa Simpson Hoover lives in Atlanta with her husband and three daughters. She grew up in Washington, D.C. graduating from The American University. She attended law school in Florida and started her career as a prosecuting attorney there. She later transitioned to civil litigation working as an insurance defense attorney for a large insurance company in Florida and Illinois. In 2006, she launched The Law Office of Lisa Simpson Hoover with offices in Chicago and Atlanta. The firm specializes in personal injury litigation. She has been practicing law for over twenty years and is licensed in five states.

In her spare time, Hoover enjoys spending time with her family, working out and consignment shopping. She is an avid snow skier, swimmer and trained classical pianist. This is her first book.

Foreword

This story of the struggle of an amazing woman to rid herself of the crutch of fake hair and accept herself fully has lessons for all of us. In particular, the message to Black girls that their own hair is the "standard of beauty" is important. As the father of three beautiful black girls this is especially impactful for me.

However, the greatest and most inspirational stories have wide and deep messages that resonate with all. This book tells the story of shedding the artificial devices that we all hide behind and embracing our true selves. Some hide behind plastic surgery; some hide behind fake hair; some hide behind fake lashes, fake eyes and fake nails; some hide behind exorbitant material things.

At its core this is a story of true and complete acceptance of self. As we love and accept ourselves completely we allow the full development of our potential. Self-love is that ultimate enlightenment from which great deeds flow. Once we love ourselves that frees us to love others in a balanced and open manner. It frees our minds to concentrate on the greater good instead of acquiring things to sooth our insecurities. As I watched my wife gradually accept her true self it only made me love her more. Her acceptance of self made her a better wife, mother and person. Self-love is a powerful thing and I am certain that this book will inspire some of you to seek and achieve it.

Robert S. Hoover, MD

Introduction – The Towel

Funny thing – all who know me as a wife, mother of three and attorney would never imagine me with fake hair. It seems inconsistent with my strong personality and quiet, unassuming confidence. Funny thing – the art of being fake is creating an image so believable that people are convinced it's authentic.

Most (but not all) little black girls fantasize and gallop around their home pretending their hair is longer than it actually is at some point in their childhood. My own daughters, despite the consistent emphasis my husband and I place on their natural beauty and censorship, are unable to withstand society's saturation through the media of a European standard of beauty.

I imagine I was 7 when I began looking at my best friend – Rachel – who happened to be Caucasian and how different our hair was. Her mom, Nancy would pick me up at our home to take me to church with Rachel and my hair would be unkempt. I recall her attempts at taking the black, wide tooth comb and hard bristle brush trying to make sense of my hair. I lowered my head in embarrassment as she unsuccessfully tried to rake through my nappy locks with puzzlement.

Over the next few years I would become obsessed with the European standard of beauty having been a huge fan of Linda Carter (Wonder Woman), Lindsey Wagner (The Bionic Women) and my biggest idol – Farrah Fawcett. I even had a shirt with Farrah's face imprinted on it. I found myself attracted to the brunette with the hour glass figure and long flowing dark brown hair. (Wonder woman) I was inspired by this blond and brunette mix with a bionic body who could run at speeds faster than a bullet and was able to capture the attention and affection of this Caucasian man – Major Steven Austin (The Bionic Man). Farrah Fawcett was the epitome of beauty for me – she was one of Charlie's Angels – great body, beautiful face, long flowing curly ringlets that cascaded down her shoulders, blue eyes, a Barbie doll perfect body, and this amazing life where she received cool assignments capturing the bad guys in exotic places.

The towel became my friend. It was my introduction into an imaginary world of long hair. It was easy and I could pretend without preparation. I would just throw any long towel I could find over my head, look in the mirror and swing my "long hair" and pretend to be Farrah Fawcettt.

Chapter 1

ELEASE and the Addiction

I was introduced to Elease at the age of fourteen. My sister made the introduction. Over the years, Elease would become the supplier of my addiction. She would later empower me with the tools to sustain my addiction for a fraction of the costs of most professional hair weaves by teaching me how to sew my own weaves. It started with braids. I would make the hour trek to Elease who at the time, lived in the northeast part of Washington, D.C. off Rhode Island Avenue. I would arrive at the large, dark Victorian style row house that had been left by her late parents feeling the chill of the early morning dusk. It started with synthetic bulk hair that I would buy from the corner Korean store.

Elease would intricately lace the foreign string into my hair as she tightly knotted ornate corn rolls. Desiring to explore styles I had seen in magazines, I transitioned to single braids using "human hair." The braids allowed me to justify my growing addiction since "braids" were socially acceptable at the time. I began to get crafty with the design opting to leave the ends unraveled as the hair cascaded around my shoulders.

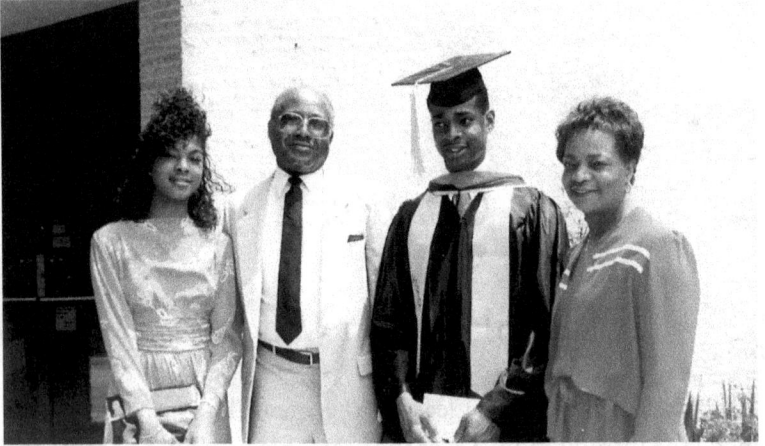

1982 photo at my brother's graduation from high school. This technique was corn rolls using wet and wavy hair that had been unraveled at the ends to achieve this look. I rationalized in my mind that this wasn't a hair weave but it was the last stage before my metamorphosis into the full fledge sew in hair weave.

Tiring of braids, Elease introduced me to hair weave extensions. She started with a small duck tail in the back of my asymmetrical cut which was the style of the 80s…. She later taught me to braid or corn roll so I could sew the tiny piece in the back of my hair myself. Proud of my sufficiency, I added a piece to the front of my hair for more length…

1985 Photo – Junior Year of high school as a model for the Saks Fifth Avenue Teen Board in Chevy Chase, Maryland. Both the front and back of my hair was a one track piece popular during the 80s. I justified this style because part of my natural hair was exposed.

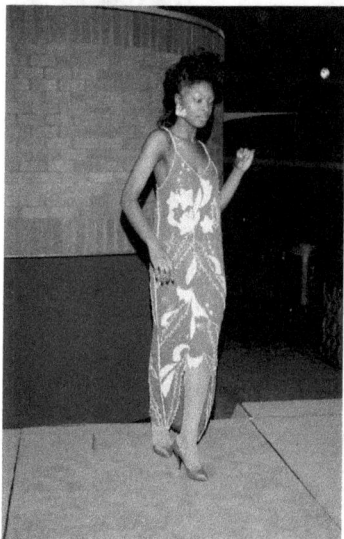

Fully equipped with the technique after months of "duck tail" pieces and bane extensions, I asked Elease to do a full hair weave after seeing a stunning up do on a hairstylist downtown. I was hooked. I would wear full and partial hair weaves throughout the remainder of high school and my freshmen year of college.

During my third year of college, I studied abroad in London. While an Elease weave got me through the first month of my study abroad experience, I was in dire need of a redo... I made the trek to the black side of town – Brixton where I bought "human hair."

With needle and thread like a junky with a syringe and heated rocks, I crept back to my home stay residence and tireless spent the three hours first corn rolling my entire head and then meticulously sewing the soft, dark brown, wavy hair into my braids. After hot curling, I was high again..... Off to the Black British Journalist Association Cocktail reception as I admired my first and successful attempt at my own hair weave... I was now empowered and would later develop the precision to create a hair weave of any style.

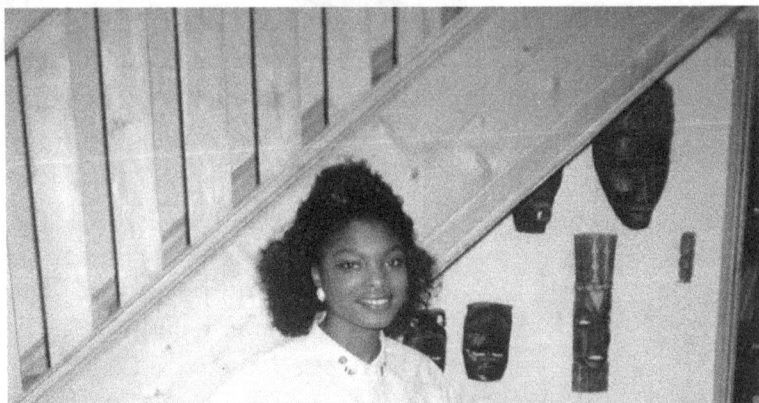

1988 photo – third year of college while studying abroad in London, England. This do-it-yourself style was a sew-in using the wet & wavy hair.

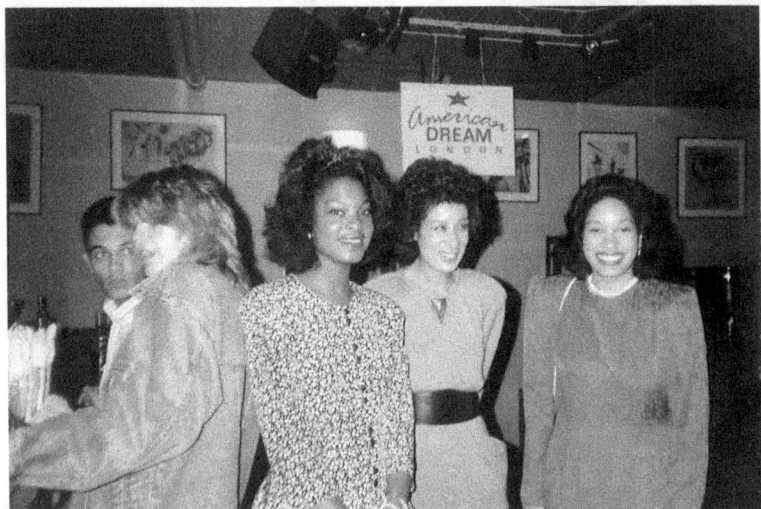

1988 Photo at Black British Journalist Association Conference in London, England. Complete sew-in using natural human hair.

Chapter 2

Maxine

I met Maxine the second semester of my second year of law school. She would become my roommate for my third and final year of law school. The University of Florida had a large Caribbean student population and their law school was no exception. Maxine was a Jamaican-born south Floridian with an aloof exterior but a warm, honest core. Throughout our year as roommates, I developed a soothing comfort around her. I could always rely on Maxine for her painfully honest yet humorous spirit. Depressed over a relationship having gone sour, I shared with Maxine that I didn't want to "burn the bridge." Maxine, with her no nonsense humor, blurted "The only bridge you are burning is his fat back that you could walk over!" she laughed.

One day as I got dressed for a date, Maxine confided that she had always been slightly envious of me because of my then Jamaican born boyfriend who courted and whisked me away for romantic candle-lit dinners - an anomaly for grant and scholarship supported black law students. She also confided that she secretly envied the popularity I enjoyed from having been the first African American female to secure a spot in the history of the coveted trial team. "But!" she exclaimed. "After I realized you wore a

hair weave," she gasped, "I didn't think you were better than me.
"   "I thought I was better than you!" she chuckled.

It was the raw purity of that statement that made me confront the perception I was creating by wearing a hair weave – one of inferiority and an unwillingness to accept my natural beauty.

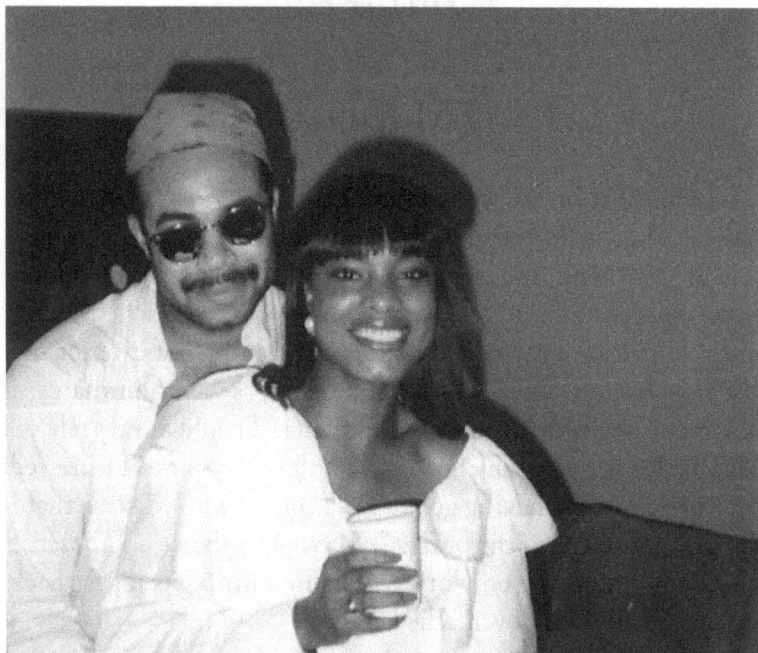

1991 photo hanging out with friend Levi from law school. Levi use to characterize any remnants of my artificial hair lying around as a "rat tail." Levi was opposed to hair weaves. In hindsight, his reluctance to commit to any serious relationship with me was due in part to my addiction.

Chapter 3

Deal Breaker

Robert and I met in the winter of 1999 in Salt Lake City, Utah. We both were attending the National Brotherhood of Skiers Annual Summit. I had mastered the art of a seamless undetectable weave with the latest in cosmetology – *bonding*. While the least healthy to my hair, bonding allowed me to blend my natural hair with the authentic human additions for a smooth wrap set style.

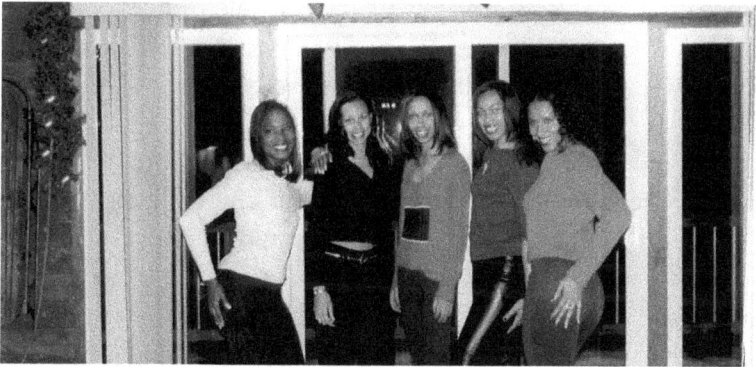

2002 photo at Copper Mountain, Colorado Ski resort with girlfriends before a night out. Everyone's hair was natural but mine. The flat wrap style utilized the bonding technique – most damaging hair weave to the natural hair follicles. Technique delivers most natural looking form of hair weave and is difficult to detect with just a basic touch of the crown of the hair.

2003 photo at Keystone, Colorado Ski resort with girlfriend before a night out. The flip style was achieved using a sew-in with

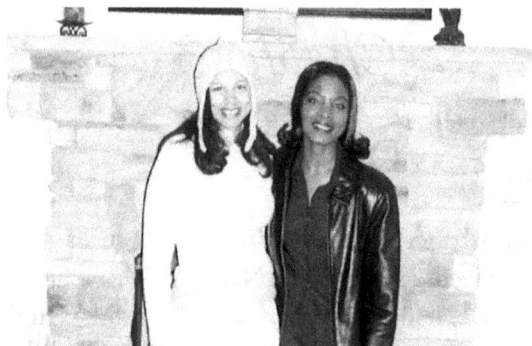

silky straight hair that gave the appearance of a natural wrap.

At the time, Robert was living in Nashville, Tennessee. I was living in Sarasota, Florida. We maintained a friendship until late 2003 when we transitioned to the same city.

While Robert had discovered the weave before 2003, the weave remain undetected long enough for him to develop a deep fondness for his soon to be wife. He would later reveal that his ignorance was due, in part, to his misconceptions about the lengths of weaves. My weave was worn modestly with the shortest length a bob extending to my chin and the longest cascading just below my collar bone.

In January of 2004, Robert and I began talking about spending our lives together. In June of 2004 he proposed. A month later, what seemed like an emotionally charged debate about the weave, became a *Deal Breaker*.

Robert exclaimed the weave was unnatural and an abomination to my natural beauty. I emphatically maintained that in light of my insecurity about my hair, I was entitled to create an image that made me comfortable and confident.

After several weeks, we arrived at a compromise. I would wear my natural hair with no addition six months out of the year.

Chapter 4

On the Fence or My Crutch?

Robert and I came to an agreement on the eve of our wedding. I would wear the hair weave only six months out of the year. I figured I'd get an early start on my end of the agreement so on our Wedding day – October 9, 2004, I went completely natural. No additions. I wore my hair pinned in a bun.

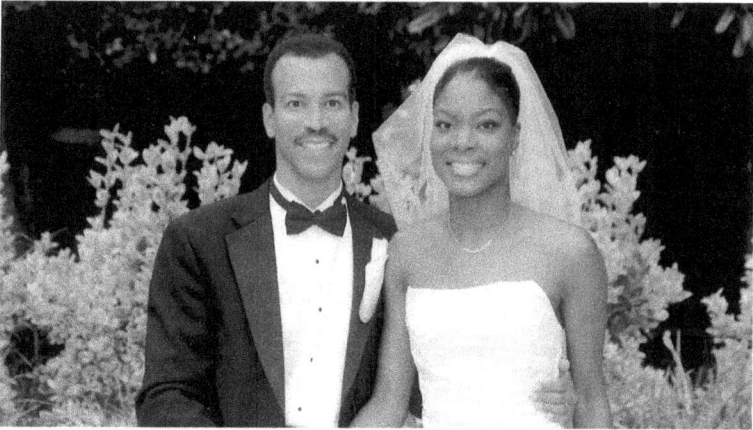

Photo of our wedding day of October 9, 2004. I decided to abandon all things artificial sans fake eye lashes.

After our honeymoon, I decided to disband the full blown hair weave and transition to wearing my hair in a ponytail with an artificial piece. It was difficult for me to completely part with hairweave so the fake ponytail gave me comfort. I could hide behind it. No one would know what my hair looked like. No one would know it wasn't mine. It would be the perfect length as to avoid any attention. It would barely touch my shoulder. I wore the ponytail piece from November of 2005 to February of 2008 – The Wedding.

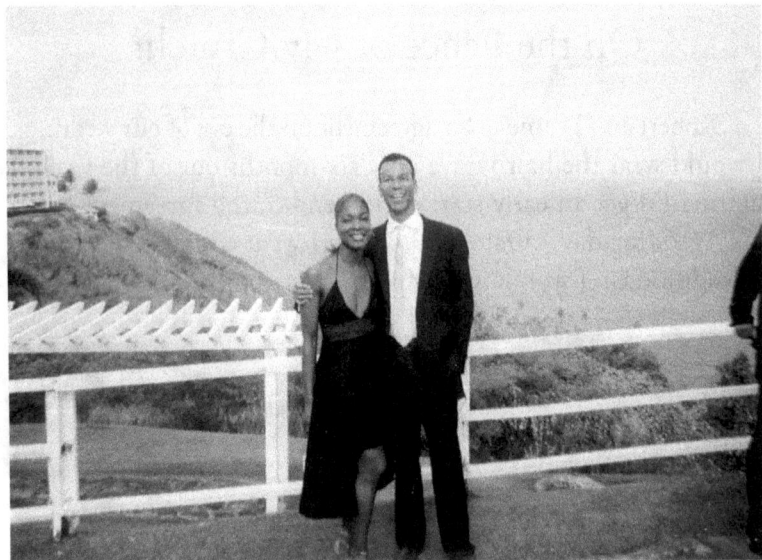

At a friends wedding in Puerto Rico. On the fence with an artificial pony tail that is natural looking.

Chapter 5

The Evolution

It was the Who's Who of Weddings in the close knit Hyde Park Community that my husband and I had settled into. A prominent middle-aged physician at The University of Chicago, and close colleague of my husband was finally tying the knot.

It was a winter wedding at the Rockefeller Chapel in Hyde Park. A full length black mink coat with my hair off my head would cover my sleek, skinny slacks, black satin stilettos and purple tunic - an appropriately elegant yet understated presence.

The wedding went off without a hitch. A cocktail reception prelude the sit down dinner. As I chatted among guests and sipped on wine, my husband approached me from the side with a discerning look. "Go to the bathroom," he said. I glared back with curiosity. "You need to fix the piece," he urged. Embarrassed while trying to maintain a slight smirk, I excused myself as I strolled into the ladies rest room. Realizing I would have to completely dismantle my hair to "fix" the "piece", I abandoned the thought and quickly left the ladies room. "No one would notice," I reassured myself.

I had to get rid of the fake "piece" I thought. My hair was simply growing longer than the piece. Unless I lengthened the "piece" it would be detected as a false addition to my hair.

With some reluctance and newfound confidence, I started wearing my hair in a ponytail. No piece. No additions.

Over the next two years, I witnessed my natural hair grow to shoulder length. I would continue to wear it in a pony tail while occasionally wearing it cascading down my shoulders to admire its length and the realization that IT WAS ALL MINE!

Chapter 6

Excuses

The top five (5) excuses we use to justify wearing hairweave and why my response is "bullshit!"

<u>Hair Growth:</u>

On average, normal black hair grows approximately 2 inches a year. Many of us never see this full growth potential due to breakage caused from chemical use, excessive heat from blow dryers and curling irons, lack of moisture, ignorance on proper hair maintenance and neglect. The harmful effects caused by mistreatment can be minimized by securing the hair in braids so there's less fuss over hair creating an environment for growth. The traditional hair weave technique where the hair is braided and the hair addition is sewn in to the braid creating a weft has often been used as an option to grow hair.

My first introduction to hair weaving began with this traditional technique. I soon realized the growth potential for my natural hair when it was secured in this hair weave. Unfortunately, my growing comfort with the softer, more easily manageable foreign locks became addictive. I became dependent on the artificial "look" achieved and dismissed any initial thoughts of resorting to a weave free style with my new hair growth.

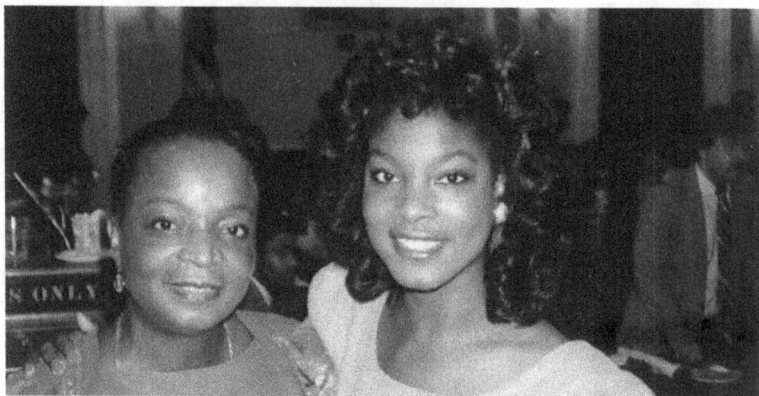

1989 Photo at Reception for Miss America Pageant Local Level Contestants with my mom. Complete sew-in using natural human hair.

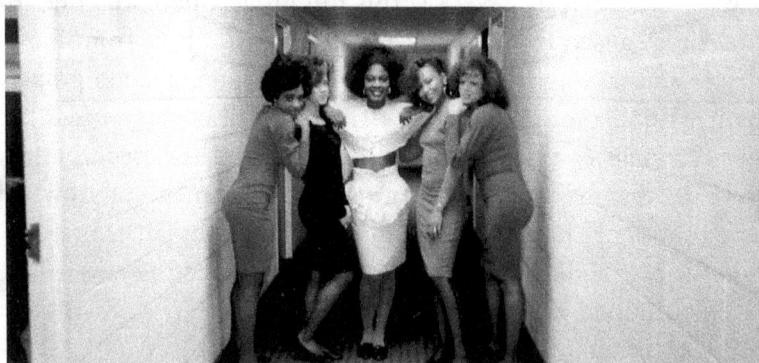

1987 Photo taken in my dormitory at American University before a night out. This big hair style was a sew-in technique using a very course texture of the wet and wavy hair brand.

Convenience:

(Lifestyle & Weather) e.g. exercise, rain. The reality is that most women who wear hair weaves, don't wear them to allow for freedom for exercise. Look at the obesity among black women in the U.S. alone. If you look at the black women working out in a gym on a regular basis or the ones whose bodies are consistent with their regular exercise pattern, you'll find they wear their hair in a natural state (twists, locks, short crop fro, short crop pixie, pony tail or wrap).

Versatility:

Different styles. This is simply an over perpetuated myth! Typically, in the instant of a hair weave, you are limited to one or two styles because of the grain direction of the hair weave to avoid detecting the root of the weave. Natural styles offer much more versatility for e.g. twists, bantu knots, wrap, wet set, pony tail (chic); updo; french roll.

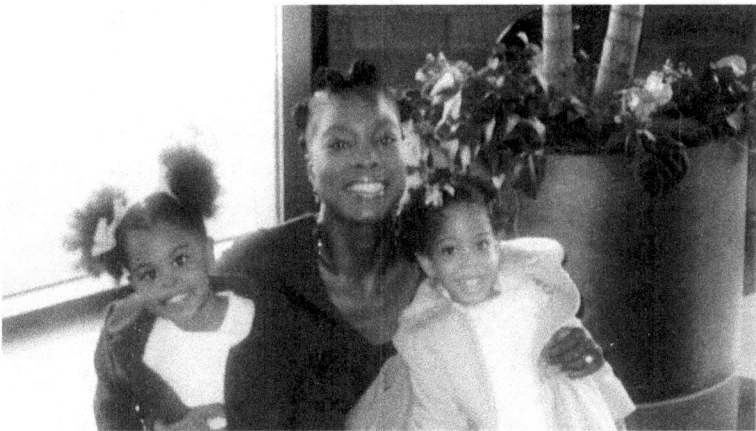

Transition:

I'm in transition from a perm to natural. My response. "Cut the shit off!"

The transition from perm to natural hair can first be a difficult choice and a process fraught with trial, error and patience. Soft, silky roots are now coarse and brittle. Proper maintenance of the roots during the grow-out process requires a balance of moisture and regular maintenance. Often unfamiliar and ignorant of our natural hair texture, black women find themselves unable to maintain a style during this transition without the use of excessive heat to the root (if continuing to wear a pressed style) or difficulty combing through the root if maintaining a natural style during the grow out. Hair weave is an option that promotes freedom from the challenges. It essentially, allows us to be lazy and take the easy way out.

My Hair isn't Thick Enough:

For years I convinced myself that my hair was thin. A hair weave would allow for a fuller look. In reality, the harsh chemicals, excessive heat from blowing dryers and curling irons along with continued extensions and hair weave wore on my ever increasingly fragile locks perpetuating the thinning process. Freedom from artificial hair allowed my hair to breath. I began to appreciate the beauty of healthy hair achieved notwithstanding the number of hair strands on my head.

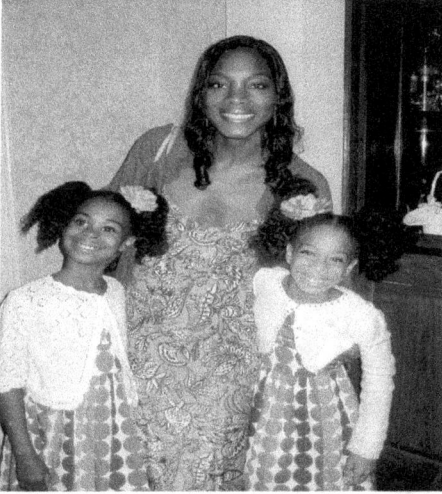

Photo taken in 2013 at a cousins' wedding with my twin daughters, Lena & Lyric. My hair was the healthiest and longest its ever been.

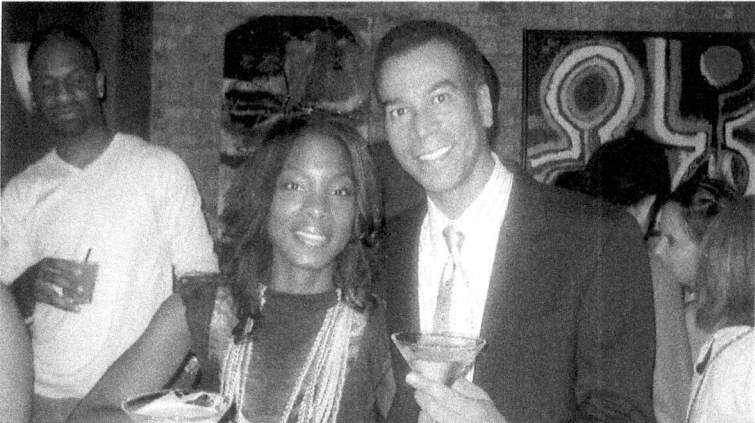

2009 Photo on a date with Robert. I am gradually becoming comfortable with my natural hair.

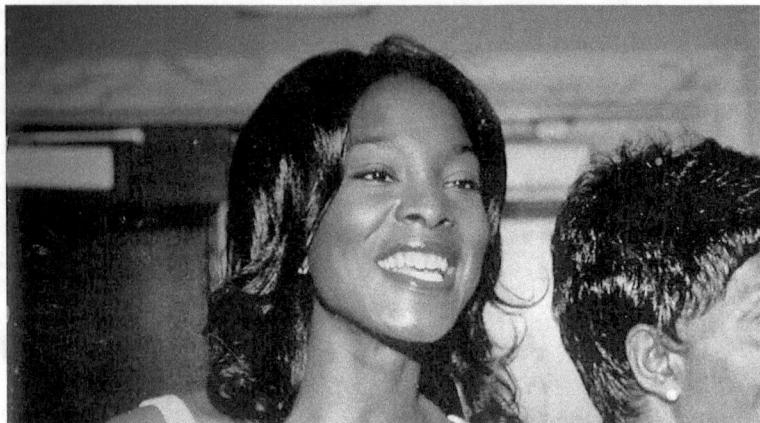

May 16th 2009 – Celebrating with my mom at her and my dad's 50th wedding anniversary further becoming comfortable being all me.

Chapter 7

The Facts – The Truth about the Harmful Affects of Weave on the Hair Growth Process

The biggest moneymaker in the hair business is artificial hair. Black women can spend six to eight hours getting their hair braided into tiny sections. Stylists then delicately attach tracks of hair -- which can be simple extensions or full wigs -- to the braids.

Women who wear weaves stop by the salon for regular washes, conditioning and tightening, but the real expense lies with the hair itself. Women spend thousands of dollars a year on weaves -- and even put them on layaway.

Much of the hair used for creating extensions for black women comes from India. It is actually one of India's largest exports behind software. At a Hindu temple, more than 10 million people -- most of them poor -- sacrifice their hair to God in a religious ceremony. In India, hair is considered a vanity, and removing hair is considered an act of self-sacrifice.

The money made at this temple is second only to the Vatican. The hair collected here is auctioned off to exporters who distribute it around the world. Once cut, the sacrificed hair is processed and sold to hair dealers around the world who, in turn, sell it to local dealers who, in turn, sell it to salons and hair vendors.

Lace Front Weave

Lace front weaves are wigs or weaves that have a small piece of mesh attached to the front that you apply to your head, giving the illusion of a hairline. Lace front weaves and wigs come in a variety of hair and textures.

The problem has always been the adhesive directly applied to the hair, scalp and skin, which poses a serious problem. Because of this, many cosmetologist have reverted to using plastic caps, stocking caps and paper strips to cover the hair which is not effective. Plastic caps cause moisture build up. Stocking caps eliminate proper circulation to the scalp and paper strips hold heat and does not stay in place.

Bonding
(Hair gluing products, bonding glue,
gold bond liquid, and ultra bonding glue.)

Hair bonding involves attaching additional strands of hair to your natural hair. The additional hair that is used may be synthetic or human. The synthetic hair can be made of many different types of synthetic fibers, and is usually cheaper than human hair, but does not last as long. It tends to get tangled a lot more than real hair, and also has a tendency to become very frizzy. Styling options are also limited, as certain techniques such as heating are not suitable for synthetic hair.

The problem with hair bonding is that the additional hair, whether synthetic or real, needs to be attached to your natural hair. This means using some kind of adhesive, which can be harmful for your hair and scalp. The chemicals used always pose the risks that your scalp or hair will react to them.

More harmful, exposure of your hair to the bonding solution for an extended period of time poses long-term damage to the hair shaft. Some users of this technique rationalize that getting rid of the bonded hair within a month prevents the long term damage. However, this means you are going through an expense for just a couple of weeks, and in any case, removing the extensions can also damage your natural hair.

Another way that gluing or bonding in a hair weave can damage African American hair is when the glue becomes stuck in the scalp. This can cause hair to come off with the weave, even if you have tried to wash the glue out of the hair. Sometimes to remove the glue entirely, it is necessary to cut the real hair, which is counterproductive.

A glue-in weave also damages African American hair over the long term because you cannot wash a weave that has been glued in, versus one that has been sewn in. Not washing your hair will leave your hair dirty, breakage will occur and the end result will be unhealthy hair.

The Sew In

A sew-in weave is a type of <u>hair extension</u> that is typically done at beauty salons where either real or synthetic human hair is sewn onto small, tightly woven braids against the scalp. In most cases, a sew-in weave will last for at least three months before it must be taken out.

A sew in takes anywhere from two to four hours to put in. It takes time to braid the existing hair against the scalp (corn roll) and then sew in the new hair.

While the Sew In appears the least harmful to the natural hair tress because there is no use of harmful chemicals and the hair appears to grow while in this weave, it is arguably more harmful over the long term to hair. Any artificial coverage of our natural hair is like putting a pillow case over a babies head. It eventually dies from suffocation because he or she is unable to breathe. Similarly, our natural hair needs air to breathe. Lack of oxygen to the hair shaft interferes with the growth of a healthy head of hair – from the root extending to the ends. Gradually, over time, the extended wear of a sew in leaves hair dry and thin. From personal experience, I witnessed my hair grow for the years that I wore a sew in weave BUT, my hair was gravely thin as a result over the years.

Chapter 8

Why Little Black Girls can't
Wear Braids with Extensions

It's subtle stuff that puts girls on the road to getting their identity from how they look, which as they get older will be increasingly defined as hot and sexy. You see it starting with the Disney princesses. Girlhood *is* different today. Its more commercialized (companies spent $100 million in advertising to kids in 1983; today they spend almost $17 *billion*), more girly (nearly everything manufactured for girls from birth is screamingly, irritatingly, blindingly pink and increasingly sexualized.

What's sexy about a little girl in a pink princess costume? "Sexy" is not the same thing as *sexualized*. Sexualization is not only imposing sexuality on children before they're ready and viewing girls as sexual objects, but also valuing a girl for her appearance over her other attributes like her personality, character, intellect and talents.

While "Princesses are just a phase," they mark a girl's "first foray into the mainstream culture. What was the first thing that society told her about being a girl? Not that she was competent, strong, creative, or smart but that every little girl wants or should want to be the fairest of them all.

The more a girl is exposed to girly-girl culture that emphasize color of skin, eyes and length of hair, the more vulnerable she is to depression, eating disorders, distorted body image, and risky sexual behavior. One study focusing on college girls show just two commercials with stereotyped portrayals of women. One, a girl raving about acne medicine and another of a woman thrilled with a brownie mix. The women shown the ads expressed less interest in math- and science-related careers afterward than girls who had not been shown the ads. In America, the average child watches an estimated 40,000 ads a year.

Just as marijuana is often associated with a gateway drug to more addictive ones, marketing aimed at little girls is a gateway to inferiority, insecurity, low self-esteem and a desire to achieve a more European form of beauty.

Unfortunately, when we expose our little girls to hair extensions at a young age, there's a message we send. The length of your hair is important. It equates beauty with length and texture rather than natural authenticity. We are training our little girls that buying and affixing artificial foreign tresses to our head is makes you beautiful.

So how do you keep your little girl from becoming *that* girl, when the line between good femme fun and aggressive, targeted consumerism is so faint? With little black girls, its no artificial hair or extensions that detract from their natural beauty.

Chapter 9

Love Yourself Inside Out
Plant the <u>SEAD</u>

The acronym **SEAD** stands for Sleep, Exercise, Attitude and Diet.

Sleep

Statistics reveal that sleep is a vital component of good health as is diet and exercise. Studies show increased exercise performance based on proper sleep. Similarly, the statistics revealed longer, deeper sleep derived from exercising on a regular basis. Weight loss has also been linked to proper sleep while weight gain has been linked to inadequate sleep. I recommend eight (8). The benefits of sleep include (a) allowing body to heal itself of stresses and fatigue of the day (b) more mental clarity and focus (c) balanced metabolism (d) positive attitude and increased energy for exercise and fitness.

Exercise

The overall health benefits of exercise makes common sense. They include (a) weight monitoring (b) improved emotional state

(c) reduced stress (d) greater likelihood of balanced sleep patterns (e) increased metabolism (f) increased self esteem and positive attitude (g) mental alertness.

Attitude and Authenticity

BBB – Black - Brilliant and Beautiful – Embrace by BELIEVING and LIVING it daily. What does this mean?

To counter the subtle impact of society's emphasis on a European form of beauty, my husband and I created the Brilliant, Black & Beautiful mantra that gets reinforced on a daily basis with our three daughters. We first censored any exposure to television or film that perpetuates a European form of beauty. We encourage them to embrace their authentic, God-given natural beauty – the color of their skin, the unique texture of their hair and the rounds and curves of their body or lack therof. This is further emphasized by daily compliments about their inner and exterior beauty. Black history material including books, comics and magazines are encouraged. Film exposure is marked by colorful, poignant portrayals of strong African American heroines, prince and princess, kings and queens. It is our hope that with early intervention, we will plant seeds that will take root as our daughters enter adolescent and maturation. At that stage and earlier, black girls are bombarded with the poison that society feeds about a European form of beauty.

Authenticity comes from examining and appreciating ones inner and exterior beauty in its natural unmodified state. <u>Here is my (6) ingredient recipe for achieving the BBB (</u>Black Brilliant Beautiful<u>) Attitude</u>.

Hobbies – Cultivate a hobby e.g. sports or arts based and work towards perfecting it. Over time, a sense of confidence in being passionate about something will build heightened self esteem.

Family Roots & Black History Heritage – Sense of Pride. Educate yourself about your family genealogy and America's black history heritage. Knowledge and enlightenment about the struggles, strength, fortitude of our ancestors generates pride and an invincibility that all things are achievable. In 2009, I researched my family tree on my mother's side and discovered an ancestral line dating back to the late 1700s. With my research, I was able to pull from census records marriage licenses for four generations dating back to the mid 1800s. The framed license certificates are prominently displayed in our home as a representation of the commitment to marriage my parents, grandparents, great grandparents and great great grand parents had to the institution of marriage. This fills me with pride and an increased resolve to commit to my marriage. Pride in wanting to maintain the sanctity of my marriage.

Exposure to the Arts. Statistics reveal that both exposure and arts immersion builds self esteem, social skills and a star attitude. As a child of the performing arts, I became comfortable in my skin by developing my dramatic skills on stage. The accolades from accomplishing a play increased my self confidence and made me feel like a star. Having trained fourteen years as a classical pianist allowed me to exude confidence that transcended race and economics.

Identify your Strengths and Cultivate them. Recognizing your personal value to society is the ultimate ego booster!

Positive Role Models with Positive Self Image. Identify positive role models in your life, on television, magazines, internet or media e.g. teacher, mentor, parent, relative, politician, friend or clergy. Envision their positive characters in your self portrait and embody those characteristics while developing your own unique positive traits.

Diet

Three meals a day. Start w/ breakfast; include high fiber diet. Moderate or minimize caffeine intake, alcohol, sweets, soda, chips, high cholesterol, high fat and high carbohydrates. Instead increase the intake of fruits, vegetables, whole grains, nuts including beans, broccoli, brown rice, quinoa. Keep animal products e.g. meat, chicken, pork, eggs , dairy & animal fat based oils to a minimum but favor foods with a low glycemic index. Instead of eggs and bacon for breakfast, opt for old fashioned oatmeal with cinnamon and fruit and rye toast. Eliminate or keep to a minimum fast food options which have been historically known on a consistent basis to cause obesity. If dining out, think international. In Mediterranean countries, Asia, Africa and Latin America, the traditional dietary staples are grains, vegetables, legumes and fruits. All these regions have historically had much lower rates of diabetes, high blood pressure, high cholesterol and obesity. When you choose the best of what these cuisines have to offer, dinner out can be both healthy and delicious.

Chapter 10

Just Do You – The Story of Daniel

In the book of Daniel in the Bible, God reveals that he gives us the strength to stand firm in him as we serve.

Daniel was from Judah but came under the reign of Babylon. He, along with other Israelites from the royal family and of nobility, was appointed to serve in the king's palace. They were to be trained for three years and after that they were to enter the king's service. They were given new names but Daniel resolved not to defile himself with the royal food and wine. He insisted that he subsist on nothing but vegetables to eat, and water to drink later proving he was stronger in every matter of wisdom and understanding than any of those who resorted to the royal food and wine.

Throughout his captivity in Babylon, Daniel showed great distinction in embracing his uniqueness in standing firm in his convictions.

Daniel was thrown in the lion's den at the request of King Nebuchadnezzar for refusing to worship false gods. Daniel stood firm in his conviction that he had one God – his lord and savior, Jesus Christ – son of the almighty God in heaven above. Although thrown into the lions' den, Daniel persevered and was spared the lions' wrath. He was unharmed! It was clear that God took care of his children.

The story of Daniel is an example of standing firm as a role model. Avoid succumbing to   societies perceptions of beauty. Just Do You as Daniel did! Embrace the God Given You!